The Best Mediterranean Dinner Recipes

Delicious Mediterranean Dinners

Sommario

Introduction

Dinner is always the most romantic time of the day, where we get together with friends, family or the person we love most.

What could be better than a Mediterranean style dinner to surprise everyone?

That's why I thought of this book, which encapsulates all the origins of the Mediterranean basin with wonderful flavors.

These recipes invented and enjoyed since ancient times are now at your disposal.

But let's start cooking right away, prepare your apron and go to the kitchen..enjoy

Dinner Recipes

Broiled Herb Sole With Cauliflower Mashed Potatoes

Servings: 4

Cooking Time: 16 Minutes

Ingredients:

- 12 ounces cauliflower florets, cut into 1-inch pieces

- 1 (12-ounce) Yukon Gold potato, cut into ¾-inch pieces (do not peel)

- 2 tablespoons olive oil

- ¼ teaspoon kosher salt

- 2 teaspoons olive oil, plus more to grease the pan

- 3 tablespoons chopped parsley

- 3 tablespoons chopped fresh dill

- 1 tablespoon freshly squeezed lemon juice

- ½ teaspoon chopped garlic

- 1¼ pounds boneless, skinless sole or tilapia

- ¼ teaspoon kosher salt

- 4 lemon wedges, for serving

Directions:

1. TO MAKE THE CAULIFLOWER MASHED POTATOES

2. Pour enough water into a saucepan that it reaches ½ inch up the side of the pan. Turn the heat to high and bring the water to a boil. Add the cauliflower and potatoes, and cover the pan. Steam for 10 minutes or until the veggies are very tender.

3. Drain the vegetables if water remains in the pan. Transfer the veggies to a large bowl and add the olive oil and salt. Taste and add an additional pinch of salt if you need it.

4. Once the veggies have cooled, scoop ¾ cup of cauliflower mashed potatoes into each of containers.

5. TO MAKE THE SOLE

6. Preheat the oven to the high broiler setting. Line a sheet pan with foil and lightly grease the pan with oil or cooking spray.

7. Mix the oil, parsley, dill, lemon juice, and garlic in a small bowl. Pat the fish with paper towels to remove excess moisture and place on the lined sheet pan. Sprinkle the salt over the fish, then spread the herb mixture over the fish. Broil for about 6 minutes or until the fish is flaky. If your fish is very thin, broil for 5 minutes.

8. When everything has cooled, place one quarter of the fish in each of the 4 cauliflower containers. Serve with lemon wedges.

9. STORAGE: Store covered containers in the refrigerator for up to 4 days.

Nutrition Info:Per Serving: Total calories: 291; Total fat: 11g; Saturated fat: 1g; Sodium: 423mg; Carbohydrates: 20g; Fiber: 2g; Protein: 29g

Citrus Poached Lovely Salmon

Servings: 4

Cooking Time: 40 Minutes

Ingredients:

- 6 cups water

- ½ cup freshly squeezed lemon juice

- Juice of 1 lime

- Zest of 1 lime

- 1 sweet onion, thinly sliced

- 1 cup celery leaves, coarsely chopped

- 1 tablespoon fresh dill, chopped

- 1 tablespoon fresh thyme, chopped

- 2 dried bay leaves

- ½ teaspoon black peppercorns

- ½ teaspoon sea salt

- 1 (24 ounce salmon side, skinned and deboned, cut into 4 pieces

Directions:

1. Take a large saucepan and place it over medium-high heat

2. Stir water, lemon, lime juice, lem0on juice, lime zest, onion, celery, greens, thyme, dill and bay leaves

3. Strain the liquid through fine mesh sieve, discard any solids

4. Pour strained poaching liquid into large skillet over low heat

5. Bring to a simmer

6. Add fish and cover skillet, poach for 10 minutes until opaque

7. Remove salmon from liquid and serve

8. Enjoy!

9. Meal Prep/Storage Options: Store in airtight containers in your fridge for 1-3 days.

Nutrition Info: Calories: 248;Fat: 11g;Carbohydrates: 4g;Protein: 34g

Bean Lettuce Wraps

Servings: 4

Cooking Time: 20 Minutes

Ingredients:

- 8 Romaine lettuce leaves

- ½ cup Garlic hummus or any prepared hummus

- ¾ cup chopped tomatoes

- 15 ounce can great northern beans, drained and rinsed

- ½ cup diced onion

- 1 tablespoon extra virgin olive oil

- ¼ cup chopped parsley

- ¼ teaspoon black pepper

Directions:

1. Set a skillet on top of the stove range over medium heat.

2. In the skillet, warm the oil for a couple of minutes.

3. Add the onion into the oil. Stir frequently as the onion cooks for a few minutes.

4. Combine the pepper and tomatoes and cook for another couple of minutes. Remember to stir occasionally.

5. Add the beans and continue to stir and cook for 2 to 3 minutes.

6. Turn the burner off, remove the skillet from heat, and add the parsley.

7. Set the lettuce leaves on a flat surface and spread 1 tablespoon of hummus on each leaf.

8. Divide the bean mixture onto the leaves.

9. Spread the bean mixture down the center of the leaves.

10. Fold the leaves by starting lengthwise on one side.

11. Fold over the other side so the leaf is completely wrapped.

12. Serve and enjoy!

Nutrition Info: calories: 211, fats: 8 grams, carbohydrates: 28 grams, protein: 10 grams.

Greek Chicken Shish Kebab

Servings: 6

Cooking Time: 10 Minutes

Ingredients:

- ¼ cup olive oil

- ¼ cup lemon juice

- ¼ cup white vinegar

- 2 garlic cloves, minced

- 1 teaspoon ground cumin

- 1 teaspoon dried oregano

- ½ teaspoon dried thyme

- ¼ teaspoon salt

- ¼ teaspoon ground black pepper

- 2 pounds boneless and skinless chicken breasts, cut up into 1½inch pieces

- 6 wooden skewers

- 2 large green or red bell peppers, cut up into 1inch pieces

- 12 cherry tomatoes

- 12 fresh mushrooms

Directions:

1. In a large bowl, whisk in olive oil, vinegar, garlic, lemon juice, cumin, thyme, oregano, salt, and black pepper. Mix well.

2. Add the chicken to the bowl and coat it thoroughly by tossing it.

3. Cover the bowl with plastic wrap, refrigerate, and allow it to marinate for 2 hours.

4. Soak your wooden skewers in water for about 30 minutes.

5. Preheat grill to medium-high heat and lightly oil the grate.

6. Remove the chicken from your marinade and shake off any extra liquid.

7. Discard the remaining marinade.

8. Thread pieces of chicken with bits of onion, bell pepper, cherry tomatoes, and mushrooms alternating between them.

9. Cook on grill for 10 minutes each side until browned on all sides.

10. Chill, place to containers.

11. Pre-heat before eating. Enjoy!

Nutrition Info:Per Serving: Calories: 183, Total Fat: 9.8 g, Saturated Fat: 1.4 g, Cholesterol: 22 mg, Sodium: 141 mg, Total Carbohydrate: 14.1 g, Dietary Fiber: 4.4 g, Total Sugars: 8.5 g, Protein: 6 g, Vitamin D: 130 mcg, Calcium: 42 mg, Iron: 3 mg, Potassium: 821 mg

Skillet Shrimp With Summer Squash And Chorizo

Servings: 8

Cooking Time: 20 Minutes

Ingredients:

- 1 lb large shrimp or prawns, peeled and deveined, tail can remain or frozen frozen, thawed

- 7 oz Spanish Chorizo, or mild Chorizo or hot Chorizo, sliced

- Extra virgin olive oil

- Juice of 1/2 lemon

- 1 summer squash, halved then sliced, half moons

- 1 small hot pepper such as jalapeno pepper, optional

- 1/2 medium red onion, sliced

- Fresh parsley for garnish

- 3/4 tsp smoked paprika

- 3/4 tsp ground cumin

- 1/2 tsp garlic powder

- Salt, to taste

- Pepper, to taste

Directions:

1. Pat shrimp dry, then season with salt, pepper, paprika, cumin, and garlic powder, toss to coat, set aside

2. In a large cast iron skillet over medium-high, add the Chorizo and brown on both sides, about 4 minutes or until the Chorizo is cooked, transfer to a plate

3. In the same skillet, add a drizzle of extra virgin olive oil if needed

4. Add the summer squash, and a sprinkle of salt and pepper and sear undisturbed for about 3 to minutes on one side. turnover and sear another 2 minutes on the other side until nicely colored, transfer the squash to the plate with Chorizo

5. In the same skillet, now add a little extra virgin olive oil and tilting to make sure the bottom is well coated

6. Once heated, add the shrimp and cook, stirring frequently, until the shrimp flesh starts to turn a little pink, but still not quite fully cooked, about 3 minutes

7. Return the Chorizo and squash to the skillet, toss to combine, cook another 3 minutes or until shrimp is cooked – its pink and the tails turn a bright red

8. Transfer the shrimp skillet to a large serving platter, allow to cool

9. Distribute among the containers, store for 2-3 days

10. To Serve: Reheat on the stove for 1-2 minutes or until heated through. Squeeze 1/2 lemon on top, and sliced red onions and hot peppers.

Nutrition Info:Per Serving: Calories:192;Carbs: 4g;Total Fat: ;Protein: 17g

Shrimp & Penne

Servings: 8

Cooking Time: 35 Minutes

Ingredients:

- Penne pasta (16 oz. pkg.)

- Salt (.25 tsp.)

- Olive oil (2 tbsp.)

- Diced tomatoes (2 - 14.5 oz. cans)

- Garlic (1 tbsp.)

- Red onion (.25 cup)

- White wine (.25 cup)

- Shrimp (1 lb.)

- Grated parmesan cheese (1 cup)

Directions:

1. Dice the red onion and garlic. Peel and devein the shrimp.

2. Add salt to a large soup pot of water and set it on the stovetop to boil. Add the pasta and cook for nine to ten minutes. Drain it thoroughly in a colander.

3. Empty oil into a skillet. Warm it using the medium temperature setting.

4. Toss in the garlic and onion to sauté until they're tender.

5. Pour in the tomatoes and wine. Continue cooking for about ten minutes, stirring occasionally.

6. Fold in the shrimp and continue cooking for about five minutes or until it's opaque.

7. Combine the pasta and shrimp and top it off with the cheese to serve.

Nutrition Info: Calories: 3 ;Fat: 8.5 grams;Protein: 24.5 grams

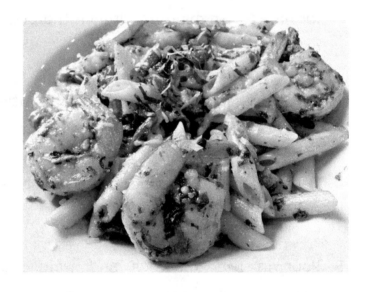

Chickpeas And Brussel Sprouts Salad

Servings: 4

Cooking Time: 10 Minutes

Ingredients:

- 1 cup roasted chickpeas. To give the dish a saltier taste, you can add sea salt.

- 4 cups kale, chopped

- 9 ounces Brussels sprouts, shredded

- 1 avocado, peeled, pitted, and cut

Directions:

1. Divide the kale and Brussels sprouts into four bowls.

2. Add the chickpeas and the avocado.

3. You can add a little sea salt and/or pepper to taste. Another tip for more taste is to drizzle a

little Vinaigrette dressing or your favorite homemade Mediterranean dressing.

Nutrition Info: calories: 337, fats: 20 grams, carbohydrates: 30 grams, protein: 12 grams.

Meat Loaf

Servings: 12

Cooking Time: 1 Hour 15 Minutes

Ingredients:

- 1 garlic clove, minced

- ½ teaspoon dried thyme, crushed

- ½ pound grass-fed lean ground beef

- 1 organic egg, beaten

- Salt and black pepper, to taste

- ¼ cup onions, chopped

- 1/8 cup sugar-free ketchup

- 2 cups mozzarella cheese, freshly grated

- ¼ cup green bell pepper, seeded and chopped

- ½ cup cheddar cheese, grated

- 1 cup fresh spinach, chopped

Directions:

1. Preheat the oven to 350 degrees F and grease a baking dish.

2. Put all the ingredients in a bowl except spinach and cheese and mix well.

3. Arrange the meat over a wax paper and top with spinach and cheese.

4. Roll the paper around the mixture to form a meatloaf.

5. Remove the wax paper and transfer the meat loaf in the baking dish.

6. Put it in the oven and bake for about 1 hour.

7. Dish out and serve hot.

8. Meal Prep Tip: Let the meat loafs cool for about 10 minutes to bring them to room temperature before serving.

Nutrition Info: Calories: 43;Carbohydrates: 8g;Protein: 40.8g;Fat: 26g ;Sugar: 1.6g;Sodium: 587mg

Couscous With Pepperoncini & Tuna

Servings: 4

Cooking Time: 20 Minutes

Ingredients:

- The Couscous:

- Chicken broth or water (1 cup)

- Couscous (1.25 cups)

- Kosher salt (.75 tsp.)

- The Accompaniments:

- Oil-packed tuna (2- 5-oz. cans)

- Cherry tomatoes (1 pint - halved)

- Sliced pepperoncini (.5 cup)

- Chopped fresh parsley (.33 cup)

- Capers (.25 cup)

- Olive oil (for serving)

- Black pepper & kosher salt (as desired)

- Lemon (1 quartered)

Directions:

1. Make the couscous in a small saucepan using water or broth. Prepare it using the medium heat temperature setting. Let it sit for about ten minutes.

2. Toss the tomatoes, tuna, capers, parsley, and pepperoncini into a mixing bowl.

3. Fluff the couscous when done and dust using the pepper and salt. Spritz it using the oil and serve with the tuna mix and a lemon wedge.

Nutrition Info: Calories: 226;Protein: 8 grams;Fat: 1 gram

Tilapia With Avocado & Red Onion

Servings: 4

Cooking Time: 15 Minutes

Ingredients:

- Olive oil (1 tbsp.)

- Sea salt (.25 tsp.)

- Fresh orange juice (1 tbsp.)

- Tilapia fillets (four 4 oz. - more rectangular than square)

- Red onion (.25 cup)

- Sliced avocado (1)

- Also Needed: 9-inch pie plate

Directions:

1. Combine the salt, juice, and oil to add into the pie dish. Work with one fillet at a time. Place it in the dish and turn to coat all sides.

2. Arrange the fillets in a wagon wheel-shaped formation. (Each of the fillets should be in the center of the dish with the other end draped over the edge.

3. Place a tablespoon of the onion on top of each of the fillets and fold the end into the center. Cover the dish with plastic wrap, leaving one corner open to vent the steam.

4. Place in the microwave using the high heat setting for three minutes. It's done when the center can be easily flaked.

5. Top the fillets off with avocado and serve.

Nutrition Info: Calories: 200;Protein: 22 grams;Fat: 11 grams

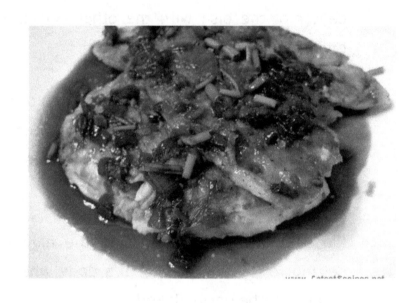

www.LatestRecipes.net

36

Baked Salmon With Dill

Servings: 4

Cooking Time: 15 Minutes

Ingredients:

- Salmon fillets (4- 6 oz. portions - 1-inch thickness)

- Kosher salt (.5 tsp.)

- Finely chopped fresh dill (1.5 tbsp.)

- Black pepper (.125 tsp.)

- Lemon wedges (4)

Directions:

1. Warm the oven in advance to reach 350° Fahrenheit.

2. Lightly grease a baking sheet with a misting of cooking oil spray and add the fish. Lightly spritz

the fish with the spray along with a shake of salt, pepper, and dill.

3. Bake it until the fish is easily flaked (10 min..)

4. Serve with lemon wedges.

Nutrition Info: Calories: 2;Protein: 28 grams;Fat: 16 grams

Steak And Veggies

Servings: 6

Cooking Time: 15 Minutes

Ingredients:

- 2 lbs baby red potatoes

- 16 oz broccoli florets

- 2 tbsp olive oil

- 3 cloves garlic, minced

- 1 tsp dried thyme

- Kosher salt, to taste

- Freshly ground black pepper, to taste

- 2 lbs (1-inch-thick) top sirloin steak, patted dry

Directions:

1. Preheat oven to broil

2. Lightly oil a baking sheet or coat with nonstick spray

3. In a large pot over high heat, boil salted water, cook the potatoes until parboiled for 12-15 minutes, drain well

4. Place the potatoes and broccoli in a single layer onto the prepared baking sheet

5. Add the olive oil, garlic and thyme, season with salt and pepper, to taste and then gently toss to combine

6. Season the steaks with salt and pepper, to taste, and add to the baking sheet in a single layer

7. Place it into oven and broil until the steak is browned and charred at the edges, about 4-5

minutes per side for medium-rare, or until the desired doneness

8. Distribute the steak and veggies among the containers. Store in the fridge for up to 3 days

9. To Serve: Reheat in the microwave for 1-2 minutes. Top with garlic butter and enjoy

Nutrition Info:Per Serving: Calories:460;Total Fat: 24g;Total Carbs: 24g;Fiber: 2.6g;Protein: 37g

Lentil And Roasted Carrot Salad With Herbs And Feta

Servings: 4

Cooking Time: 25 Minutes

Ingredients:

- ¾ cup brown or green lentils

- 3 cups water

- 1 pound baby carrots, halved on the diagonal

- 2 teaspoons olive oil, plus 2 tablespoons

- ½ teaspoon kosher salt, divided

- 1 teaspoon garlic powder

- 1 cup packed parsley leaves, chopped

- ½ cup packed cilantro leaves, chopped

- ¼ cup packed mint leaves, chopped

- ½ teaspoon grated lemon zest

- 4 teaspoons freshly squeezed lemon juice

- ¼ cup crumbled feta cheese

Directions:

1. Preheat the oven to 400°F. Line a sheet pan with a silicone baking mat or parchment paper.

2. Place the lentils and water in a medium saucepan and turn the heat to high. As soon as the water comes to a boil, turn the heat to low and simmer until the lentils are firm yet tender, 10 to minutes (see tip). Drain and cool.

3. While the lentils are cooking, place the carrots on the sheet pan and toss with 2 teaspoons of oil, ¼ teaspoon of salt, and the garlic powder. Roast the carrots in the oven until firm yet tender, about 20 to 25 minutes. Cool when done.

4. In a large bowl, mix the cooled lentils, carrots, parsley, cilantro, mint, lemon zest, lemon juice, feta, the remaining 2 tablespoons of oil, and the remaining ¼ teaspoon of salt. Add more lemon juice and/or salt to taste if needed.

5. Place 1¼ cups of the mixture in each of 4 containers.

6. STORAGE: Store covered containers in the refrigerator for up to 5 days.

Nutrition Info:Per Serving: Total calories: 2; Total fat: 12g; Saturated fat: 3g; Sodium: 492mg; Carbohydrates: 31g; Fiber: 13g; Protein: 12g

Cinnamon Squash Soup

Servings: 6

Cooking Time: 1 Hour

Ingredients:

- 1 small butternut squash, peeled and cut up into 1-inch pieces

- 4 tablespoons extra-virgin olive oil, divided

- 1 small yellow onion

- 2 large garlic cloves

- 1 teaspoon salt, divided

- 1 pinch black pepper

- 1 teaspoon dried oregano

- 2 tablespoons fresh oregano

- 2 cups low sodium chicken stock

- 1 cinnamon stick

- ½ cup canned white kidney beans, drained and rinsed

- 1 small pear, peeled and cored, chopped up into ½ inch pieces

- 2 tablespoons walnut pieces

- ¼ cup Greek yogurt

- 2 tablespoons freshly chopped parsley

Directions:

1. Preheat oven to 425 degrees F.

2. Place squash in bowl and season with a ½ teaspoon of salt and tablespoons of olive oil.

3. Spread the squash onto a roasting pan and roast for about 25 minutes until tender.

4. Set aside squash to let cool.

5. Heat remaining 2 tablespoons of olive oil in a medium-sized pot over medium-high heat.

6. Add onions and sauté until soft.

7. Add dried oregano and garlic and sauté for 1 minute and until fragrant.

8. Add squash, broth, pear, cinnamon stick, pepper, and remaining salt.

9. Bring mixture to a boil.

10. Once the boiling point is reached, add walnuts and beans.

11. Reduce the heat and allow soup to cook for approximately 20 minutes until flavors have blended well.

12. Remove the cinnamon stick.

13. Use an immersion blender and blend the entire mixture until smooth.

14. Add yogurt gradually while whisking to ensure that you are getting a very creamy soup.

15. Season with some additional salt and pepper if needed.

16. Garnish with parsley and fresh oregano.

17. Enjoy!

Nutrition Info:Per Serving: Calories: 197, Total Fat: 11.6 g, Saturated Fat: 1.7 g, Cholesterol: 0 mg, Sodium: 264 mg, Total Carbohydrate: 20.2 g, Dietary Fiber: 7.1 g, Total Sugars: 4.3 g, Protein: 6.1 g, Vitamin D: 0 mcg, Calcium: 103 mg, Iron: 3 mg, Potassium: 425 mg

Creamy Chicken

Servings: 2

Cooking Time: 25 Minutes

Ingredients:

- ½ small onion, chopped

- ¼ cup sour cream

- Salt and black pepper, to taste

- 1 tablespoon butter

- ¼ cup mushrooms

- ½ pound chicken breasts

Directions:

1. Heat butter in a skillet and add onions and mushrooms.

2. Sauté for about 5 minutes and add chicken breasts and salt.

3. Secure the lid and cook for about 5 more minutes.

4. Add sour cream and cook for about 3 minutes.

5. Open the lid and dish out in a bowl to serve immediately.

6. Transfer the creamy chicken breasts in a dish and set aside to cool for meal prepping. Divide them in 2 containers and cover their lid. Refrigerate for 2-3 days and reheat in microwave before serving.

Nutrition Info: Calories: 335 ;Carbohydrates: 2.9g;Protein: 34g;Fat: 20.2g;Sugar: 0.8g;Sodium: 154mg

Chicken Drummies With Peach Glaze

Servings: 4

Cooking Time: 25 Minutes

Ingredients:

- 2 pounds of chicken drummies, remove the skin

- 15 ounce can of sliced peaches, drain the juice

- ¼ cup cider vinegar

- ½ teaspoon paprika

- ¼ teaspoon black pepper

- ¼ cup honey

- 3 garlic cloves

- ¼ teaspoon sea salt

Directions:

1. Before you turn your oven on, make sure that one rack is 4 inches below the broiler element.

2. Set your oven's temperature to 500 degrees Fahrenheit.

3. Line a large baking sheet with a piece of aluminum foil.

4. Set a wire cooling rack on top of the foil.

5. Spray the rack with cooking spray.

6. Add the honey, peaches, garlic, vinegar, salt, paprika, and pepper into a blender. Mix until smooth.

7. Set a medium saucepan on top of your stove and set the range temperature to medium heat.

8. Pour the mixture into the saucepan and bring it to a boil while stirring constantly.

9. Once the sauce is done, divide it into two small bowls and set one off to the side.

10. With the second bowl, brush half of the mixture onto the chicken drummies.

11. Roast the drummies for 10 minutes.

12. Take the drummies out of the oven and switch to broiler mode.

13. Brush the drummies with the other half of the sauce from the second bowl.

14. Again, place the drummies back into the oven and set a timer for 5 minutes.

15. When the timer goes off, flip the drummies over and broil for another 3 to 4 minutes.

16. Serve the drummies with the reserved sauce and enjoy!

Nutrition Info: calories: 291, fats: 5 grams, carbohydrates: 33 grams, protein: 30 grams.

Berry Compote With Orange Mint Infusion

Servings: 8

Cooking Time: 20 Minutes

Ingredients:

- ½ cup water

- 3 orange pekoe tea bags

- 3 sprigs of fresh mint

- 1 cup fresh strawberries, hulled and halved lengthwise

- 1 cup fresh golden raspberries

- 1 cup fresh red raspberries

- 1 cup fresh blueberries

- 1 cup fresh blackberries

- 1 cup fresh sweet cherries, pitted and halved

- 1-milliliter bottle of Sauvignon Blanc

- 2/3 cup sugar

- ½ cup pomegranate juice

- 1 teaspoon vanilla

- fresh mint sprigs

Directions:

1. In a small saucepan, bring water to a boil and add tea bags and 3 mint sprigs.

2. Stir well, cover, remove from heat, and allow to stand for 10 minutes.

3. In a large bowl, add strawberries, red raspberries, golden raspberries, blueberries, blackberries, and cherries. Put to the side.

4. In a medium-sized saucepan, and add the wine, sugar, and pomegranate juice.

5. Pour the infusion (tea mixture) through a fine-mesh sieve and into the pan with wine.

6. Squeeze the bags to release the liquid, and then discard bags and mint springs.

7. Cook well until the sugar has completely dissolved; remove from heat.

8. Stir in vanilla and allow to chill for 2 hours.

9. Pour the mix over the fruits.

10. Garnish with mint sprigs and serve.

11. Enjoy!

Nutrition Info:Per Serving: Calories: 119, Total Fat: 0.3 g, Saturated Fat: 0 g, Cholesterol: 0 mg, Sodium: 3 mg, Total Carbohydrate: 31.6 g, Dietary Fiber: 5 g, Total Sugars: 26.2 g, Protein: 1.2 g, Vitamin D: 0 mcg, Calcium: 28 mg, Iron: 1 mg, Potassium: 158 mg

Quinoa Bruschetta Salad

Servings: 5

Cooking Time: 15 Minutes

Ingredients:

- 2 cups water

- 1 cup uncooked quinoa

- 1 (10-ounce) container cherry tomatoes, quartered

- 1 teaspoon chopped garlic

- 1¼ cups thinly sliced scallions, white and green parts (1 small bunch)

- 1 (8-ounce) container fresh whole-milk mozzarella balls (ciliegine), quartered

- 2 tablespoons balsamic vinegar

- 2 tablespoons olive oil

- ½ teaspoon kosher salt

- ½ cup fresh basil leaves, chiffonaded (cut into strips)

Directions:

1. Place the water and quinoa in a saucepan and bring to a boil. Cover, turn the heat to low, and simmer for minutes.

2. While the quinoa is cooking, place the tomatoes, garlic, scallions, mozzarella, vinegar, and oil in a large mixing bowl. Stir to combine.

3. Once the quinoa is cool, add it to the tomato mixture along with the salt and basil. Mix to combine.

4. Place 1⅓ cups of the mixture in each of 5 containers and refrigerate. Serve at room temperature.

5. STORAGE: Store covered containers in the refrigerator for up to days.

Nutrition Info:Per Serving: Total calories: 323; Total fat: 1; Saturated fat: 6g; Sodium: 317mg; Carbohydrates: 30g; Fiber: 4g; Protein: 14g

Zesty Lemon Parmesan Chicken And Zucchini Noodles

Servings: 2

Cooking Time: 15 Minutes

Ingredients:

- 2 packages Frozen zucchini noodle Spirals

- 1-1/2 lbs. boneless skinless chicken breast, cut into bite-sized pieces

- 1 tsp fine sea salt

- 2 tsp dried oregano

- 1/2 tsp ground black pepper

- 4 garlic cloves, minced

- 2 tbsp vegan butter

- 2 tsp lemon zest

- 2 tsp oil

- 1/3 cup parmesan

- 2/3 cup broth

- Lemon slices, for garnish

- Parsley, for garnish

Directions:

1. Cook zucchini noodles according to package instructions, drain well

2. In a large skillet over medium heat, add the oil

3. Season chicken with salt and pepper, brown chicken pieces, for about 4 minutes per side depending on the thickness, or until cooked through – Work in cook in batches if necessary

4. Transfer the chicken to a pan

5. In the same skillet, add in the garlic, and cook until fragrant about 30 seconds

6. Add in the butter, oregano and lemon zest, pour in chicken broth to deglaze making sure to scrape up all the browned bits stuck to the bottom of the pan

7. Turn the heat up to medium-high, bring sauce and chicken up to a boil, immediately lower the heat and stir in the parmesan cheese

8. Place the chicken back in pan and allow it to gently simmer for 3-4 minutes, or until sauce has slightly reduced and thickened up

9. Taste and adjust seasoning, allow the noodles to cool completely

10. Distribute among the containers, store for 2-3 days

11. To Serve: Reheat in the microwave for 1-2 minutes or until heated through. Garnish with the fresh parsley and lemon slices and enjoy!

Nutrition Info:Per Serving: Calories:633;Carbs: 4g;Total Fat: 35g;Protein: 70g

Three Citrus Sauce Scallops

Servings: 4

Cooking Time: 15 Minutes

Ingredients:

- 2 teaspoons extra virgin olive oil

- 1 shallot, minced

- 20 sea scallops, cleaned

- 1 tablespoon lemon zest

- 2 teaspoons orange zest

- 1 teaspoon lime zest

- 1 tablespoon fresh basil, chopped

- ½ cup freshly squeezed lemon juice

- 2 tablespoons honey

- 1 tablespoon plain Greek yogurt

- Pinch of sea salt

Directions:

1. Take a large skillet and place it over medium-high heat

2. Add olive oil and heat it up

3. Add shallots and Saute for 1 minute

4. Add scallops in the skillet and sear for 5 minutes, turning once

5. Move scallops to edge and stir in lemon, orange, lime zest, basil, orange juice and lemon juice

6. Simmer the sauce for 3 minutes

7. Whisk in honey, yogurt and salt

8. Cook for 4 minutes and coat the scallops in the sauce

9. Serve and enjoy!

10. Meal Prep/Storage Options: Store in airtight containers in your fridge for 1-2 days.

Nutrition **Info:**Calories: 207;Fat: 4g;Carbohydrates: 17g;Protein: 26g

Steamed Mussels Topped With Wine Sauce

Servings: 4

Cooking Time: 15 Minutes

Ingredients:

- 2 pounds mussels

- 1 tablespoon extra virgin olive oil

- 1 cup sliced onion

- 1 cup dry white wine

- ¼ teaspoon ground black pepper

- ¼ teaspoon sea salt

- 3 sliced cloves of garlic

- 2 lemon slices

- Optional: lemon wedges for serving

Directions:

1. Set a large colander in the sink and turn your water to cold.

2. Run water over the mussels, but do not let them sit in the water. If you notice any shells that are not tightly sealed or are cracked, you need to discard them. All shells need to be closed tightly.

3. Turn off the water and leave the mussels in the colander.

4. Set a large skillet on your stovetop and turn your range heat to medium-high.

5. Pour the olive oil into the skillet and allow it to heat up before you add the onion.

6. Saute the onion for 2 to 3 minutes.

7. Combine the garlic and cook the mixture for another minute while stirring continuously.

8. Pour in the wine, pepper, lemon slices, and salt. Stir the ingredients as you bring them to a boil.

9. Add the mussels and place the lid on the skillet.

10. Cook the mixture for 3 to 4 minutes or until the shells begin to open on the mussels. It will help to gently pick up the skillet and shake it a couple of times when the mussels are cooking.

11. If you notice any shells that did not open, use a spoon and discard them.

12. Scoop the mussels into a serving bowl and pour the mixture over the top.

13. If you have lemon wedges, place them on the top of the steamed mussels before serving. Enjoy!

Nutrition Info: calories: 222, fats: 7 grams, carbohydrates: 11 grams, protein: 18 grams.

Spice Potato Soup

Servings: 4-6

Cooking Time: 30 Minutes

Ingredients:

- 2 tablespoons extra virgin olive oil

- 1 large onion, chopped

- 2 garlic cloves, crushed

- 1 pound sweet potatoes, peeled and cut into medium pieces

- ½ teaspoon ground cumin

- ¼ teaspoon ground chili

- ½ teaspoon ground coriander

- ¼ teaspoon ground cinnamon

- ¼ teaspoon salt

- 2 cups chicken stock

- ¼ cup of low-fat crème Fraiche

- 2 tablespoons freshly chopped parsley

- coriander

Directions:

1. Heat olive oil in a large pan over medium-high heat.

2. Add onions and sauté until slightly browned.

3. Reduce heat to medium, add garlic, and keep cooking for 2-minutes more.

4. Add sweet potatoes and sauté for 3-minutes.

5. Add the remaining spices and season with salt.

6. Cook for 2 minutes.

7. Add stock, turn the heat up, and bring the mixture to a boil, stirring occasionally.

8. Cover and lower heat to a slow simmer.

9. Cook for 20 minutes until the potatoes are tender.

10. Remove the pan from the heat.

11. Take an immersion blender and puree the whole mixture.

12. Add a bit of water if the soup is too thick.

13. Check the soup for seasoning.

14. Ladle the soup into your jars.

15. Give a swirl of crème Fraiche.

16. Sprinkle with chopped parsley.

17. Enjoy!

Nutrition Info:Per Serving: Calories: 176, Total Fat: 8.4 g, Saturated Fat: 0.8 g, Cholesterol: 0 mg, Sodium: 362 mg, Total Carbohydrate: 24.3 g, Dietary Fiber: 3.8 g, Total Sugars: 1.7 g, Protein: 2 g, Vitamin

D: 0 mcg, Calcium: 30 mg, Iron: 1 mg, Potassium: 675 mg

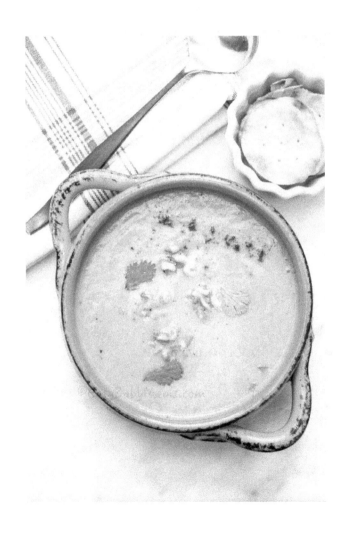

Spicy Cajun Shrimp

Servings: 2

Cooking Time: 50 Minutes

Ingredients:

- 3 cloves garlic, crushed

- 4 tablespoons butter, divided

- 2 large zucchini, spiraled

- 1 red pepper, sliced

- 1 onion, sliced

- 20-30 jumbo shrimp

- 1 teaspoon paprika

- dash cayenne pepper

- ½ teaspoon of sea salt

- dash red pepper flakes

- 1 teaspoon garlic powder

- 1 teaspoon onion powder

Directions:

1. Pass the zucchini through a spiralizer.

2. Combine the Ingredients: listed under Cajun Seasoning above.

3. Add oil and 2 tablespoons of butter to a pan and allow to heat up over medium heat.

4. Add onion and red pepper and sauté for minutes.

5. Add shrimp and cook well.

6. Place the remaining 2 tablespoons of butter in another pan and allow it to melt over medium heat.

7. Add zucchini noodles and sauté for 3 minutes.

8. Transfer the noodles to a container.

9. Top with the prepared Cajun shrimp and veggie mix.

10. Season with salt and enjoy!

Nutrition Info:Per Serving: Calories: 734, Total Fat: 24.2 g, Saturated Fat: 14.7 g, Cholesterol: 12mg, Sodium: 6703 mg, Total Carbohydrate: 29.1 g, Dietary Fiber: 7.1 g, Total Sugars: 24.9 g, Protein: 106.8 g, Vitamin D: 16 mcg, Calcium: 694 mg, Iron: 6 mg, Potassium: 1229 mg

Pan-seared Salmon

Servings: 4

Cooking Time: 20 Minutes

Ingredients:

- Salmon fillets (4 @ 6 oz. each)

- Olive oil (2 tbsp.)

- Capers (2 tbsp.)

- Pepper & salt (.125 tsp. each)

- Lemon (4 slices)

Directions:

1. Warm a heavy skillet for about three minutes using the medium heat temperature setting.

2. Lightly spritz the salmon with oil. Arrange them in the pan and increase the temperature setting to high.

77

3. Sear for approximately three minutes. Sprinkle with the salt, pepper, and capers.

4. Flip the salmon over and continue cooking for five minutes or until browned the way you like it.

5. Garnish with lemon slices and serve.

Nutrition Info: Calories: 371;Protein: 33.7 grams;Fat: 25.1 grams

Pasta Faggioli Soup

Servings: 8

Cooking Time: 1 Hour

Ingredients:

- 1 28-ounce can diced tomatoes

- 1 14-ounce can great northern beans, undrained

- 14 ounces spinach, chopped and drained

- 1 14-ounce can tomato sauce

- 3 cups chicken broth

- 1 tablespoon garlic, minced

- 8 slices bacon, cooked crisp, crumbled

- 1 tablespoon dried parsley

- 1 teaspoon garlic powder

- 1½ teaspoons salt

- ½ teaspoon ground black pepper

- ½ teaspoon dried basil

- ½ pound seashell pasta

- 3 cups water

Directions:

1. Take a large stockpot and add the diced tomatoes, spinach, beans, chicken broth, tomato sauce, water, bacon, garlic, parsley, garlic powder, pepper, salt, and basil.

2. Put it over medium-high heat and bring the mixture to a boil.

3. Immediately reduce the heat to low and simmer for 40 minutes, covered.

4. Add pasta and cook uncovered for about 10 minutes until al dente.

5. Ladle the soup into serving bowls.

6. Sprinkle some cheese on top.

7. Enjoy!

Nutrition Info:Per Serving: Calories: 23 Total Fat: 2.3 g, Saturated Fat: 0.7 g, Cholesterol: 2 mg, Sodium: 2232 mg, Total Carbohydrate: 40.6 g, Dietary Fiber: 13.1 g, Total Sugars: 6.4 g, Protein: 16.3 g, Vitamin D: 0 mcg, Calcium: 160 mg, Iron: 5 mg, Potassium: 1455 mg

Fattoush Salad

Servings: 4

Cooking Time: 10 Minutes

Ingredients:

- 2 loaves pita bread

- 3 tablespoons extra virgin olive oil

- ½ teaspoon of sumac

- salt

- pepper

- 1 heart romaine lettuce, chopped

- 1 English cucumber, chopped

- 5 Roma tomatoes, chopped

- 5 green onions, chopped

- 5 radishes, stems removed, thinly sliced

- 2 cups fresh parsley leaves, stems removed, chopped

- 1 cup fresh mint leaves, chopped

- lime juice, 1½ limes

- 1/3 bottle extra virgin olive oil

- salt

- pepper

- 1 teaspoon ground sumac

- ¼ teaspoon ground cinnamon

- scant ¼ teaspoon ground allspice

Directions:

1. Toast pita bread until crisp but not browned.

2. Heat 3 tablespoons of olive oil in a large pan over medium heat.

3. Break the toasted pita into pieces and add them to the oil.

4. Fry pita bread until browned, making sure to toss them from time to time.

5. Add salt, ½ a teaspoon of sumac, and pepper.

6. Remove the pita from the heat and place on a paper towel to drain.

7. In a large mixing bowl, combine lettuce, tomatoes, cucumber, green onions, parsley, and radish.

8. Before serving, make the lime vinaigrette by mixing all Ingredients: listed above under vinaigrette in a separate bowl.

9. Pour the vinaigrette over the Ingredients: in the other bowl and gently toss.

10. Add pita chips on top and the remaining sumac.

11. Give it a final toss and enjoy!

Nutrition Info:Per Serving: Calories: 200, Total Fat: 11.5 g, Saturated Fat: 1.7 g, Cholesterol: 0 mg, Sodium: 113 mg, Total Carbohydrate: 23.5 g, Dietary Fiber: 5.8 g, Total Sugars: 6.6 g, Protein: 5.2 g, Vitamin D: 0 mcg, Calcium: 145 mg, Iron: 6 mg, Potassium: 852 mg

Roast Chicken

Servings: 6

Cooking Time: 1 – 1 ½ Hour

Ingredients:

- fresh orange juice, 1 large orange

- ¼ cup Dijon mustard

- ¼ cup olive oil

- 4 teaspoons dried Greek oregano

- salt

- ground black pepper

- 12 potatoes, peeled and cubed

- 5 garlic cloves, minced

- 1 whole chicken

Directions:

1. Preheat oven to 375 degrees F.

2. Take a bowl and whisk in orange juice, Greek oregano, Dijon mustard, salt, and pepper. Mix well.

3. Add potatoes to the bowl and coat them thoroughly.

4. Transfer the potatoes to a large baking dish, leaving remaining juice in a bowl.

5. Stuff the garlic cloves into your chicken (under the skin).

6. Place the chicken into the bowl with the remaining juice and coat it thoroughly.

7. Transfer chicken to the baking dish, placing it on top of the potatoes.

8. Pour any extra juice on top of chicken and potatoes.

9. Bake uncovered until the thickest part of the chicken registers 160 degrees F, and the juices run clear, anywhere from 60 – minutes.

10. Remove the chicken and cover it with doubled aluminum foil.

11. Allow it to rest for 10 minutes.

12. Slice, spread over containers and enjoy!

Nutrition Info:Per Serving: Calories: 1080, Total Fat: 36.4 g, Saturated Fat: 8.8 g, Cholesterol: 325 mg, Sodium: 458 mg, Total Carbohydrate: 70.5 g, Dietary Fiber: 11.1 g, Total Sugars: 6.3 g, Protein: 16 g, Vitamin D: 0 mcg, Calcium: 120 mg, Iron: 7 mg, Potassium: 2691 mg

Chicken Eggplant

Servings: 5

Cooking Time: 40 Minutes

Ingredients:

- 3 pieces of eggplants, peeled and cut up lengthwise into ½ inch slices

- 3 tablespoons olive oil

- 6 skinless and boneless chicken breast halves, diced

- 1 onion, diced

- 2 tablespoons tomato paste

- ½ cup water

- 2 teaspoons dried oregano

- salt

- pepper

Directions:

1. Place the eggplant strips in a large pot filled with lightly salted water.

2. Allow them to soak for 30 minutes.

3. Remove the eggplant from the pot and brush thoroughly with olive oil.

4. Heat a skillet over medium heat.

5. Add eggplant and sauté for a few minutes.

6. Transfer the sautéed eggplant to a baking dish.

7. Heat a large skillet over medium heat.

8. Add chicken, onion, and sauté.

9. Stir in water and tomato paste.

10. Reduce heat to low, cover, and simmer for minutes.

11. Preheat oven to 400 degrees F.

12. Pour the chicken tomato mix over your eggplant.

13. Season with oregano, pepper, and salt.

14. Cover with aluminum foil and bake for 20 minutes.

15. Cool, place to containers and chill.

Nutrition Info:Per Serving: Calories: 319, Total Fat: 11.3 g, Saturated Fat: 1.2 g, Cholesterol: 117 mg, Sodium: 143 mg, Total Carbohydrate: 7.2 g, Dietary Fiber: 3.1 g, Total Sugars: 3.5 g, Protein: 48 g, Vitamin D: 0 mcg, Calcium: 22 mg, Iron: 2 mg, Potassium: 244 mg

Grilled Steak

Servings: 2

Cooking Time: 15 Minutes

Ingredients:

- ¼ cup unsalted butter

- 2 garlic cloves, minced

- ¾ pound beef top sirloin steaks

- ¾ teaspoon dried rosemary, crushed

- 2 oz. parmesan cheese, shredded

- Salt and black pepper, to taste

Directions:

1. Preheat the grill and grease it.

2. Season the sirloin steaks with salt and black pepper.

3. Transfer the steaks on the grill and cook for about 5 minutes on each side.

4. Dish out the steaks in plates and keep aside.

5. Meanwhile, put butter and garlic in a pan and heat until melted.

6. Pour it on the steaks and serve hot.

7. Divide the steaks in 2 containers and refrigerate for about 3 days for meal prepping purpose. Reheat in microwave before serving.

Nutrition Info: Calories: 3 ;Carbohydrates: 1.5g ;Protein: 41.4g;Fat: 23.6g;Sugar: 0g;Sodium: 352mg

Beef And Veggie Lasagna

Servings: 10

Cooking Time: 1 Hour 10 Minutes

Ingredients:

- 3 teaspoons olive oil, divided

- 1 medium zucchini, quartered lengthwise and chopped (about 1⅓ cups)

- 3 cups packed baby spinach

- 1 cup chopped yellow onion

- 1 teaspoon chopped garlic

- 8 ounces button or cremini mushrooms, finely chopped

- 1 cup shredded carrots

- 8 ounces lean (90/10) ground beef

- ½ cup dry red wine

- 1 (28-ounce) can low-sodium or no-salt-added crushed tomatoes

- 1 (15-ounce) can tomato sauce

- ¼ teaspoon kosher salt

- 1 (16-ounce) container low-fat (2%) cottage cheese

- 1 large egg

- 3 tablespoons grated Parmesan cheese

- 2 cups shredded part-skim mozzarella cheese, divided

- ½ cup fresh basil leaves, chopped

- 1 (9-ounce) box oven-ready lasagna noodles

Directions:

1. Preheat the oven to 375°F.

2. Heat 1 teaspoon of oil in a 1inch skillet over medium-high heat. When the oil is shimmering, add the zucchini and cook for 2 minutes. Add the spinach and continue to cook for 1 more minute. Remove the veggies to a plate.

3. In the same skillet, heat the remaining 2 teaspoons of oil over medium-high heat. When the oil is hot, add the onion and garlic and cook for 2 minutes. Add the mushrooms and carrots and cook for 4 more minutes. Add the ground beef and continue cooking for 4 more minutes, until the meat has browned. Add the wine and cook for 1 minute. Add the crushed tomatoes, tomato sauce, and salt, stir, and turn off the heat.

4. In a large mixing bowl, combine the cottage cheese, egg, and Parmesan, ½ cup of shredded cheese, and the basil.

5. Ladle 2 cups of sauce on the bottom of a 9-by-13-inch glass or ceramic baking dish. Place 4 noodles side by side in the pan. Layer 1 cup of

sauce, half of the veggies, and half of the cottage cheese. Repeat with 4 more noodles, 1 cup of sauce, the remaining half of the veggies, and the remaining half of the cottage cheese. Top with 4 more noodles, the remainder of the sauce, and the remaining 1½ cups of shredded cheese.

6. Cover the pan with foil, trying not to touch the foil to the cheese, and bake for 40 minutes. Remove the foil and bake for 10 to 15 more minutes, until the cheese starts to brown.

7. When the lasagna cools, cut it into 10 pieces and place 1 piece in each of 10 containers.

8. STORAGE: Store covered containers in the refrigerator for up to 5 days. Cooked lasagna freezes well and can last for up to 3 months.

Nutrition Info:Per Serving: Total calories: 321; Total fat: 11g; Saturated fat: 4g; Sodium: 680mg; Carbohydrates: 34g; Fiber: 5g; Protein: 24g

Greek Shrimp And Farro Bowls

Servings: 4

Cooking Time: 20 Minutes

Ingredients:

- 1 lb peeled and deveined shrimp

- 3 Tbsp. extra virgin olive oil

- 2 cloves garlic, minced

- 2 bell peppers, sliced thick

- 2 medium-sized zucchinis, sliced into thin rounds

- pint cherry tomatoes, halved

- ¼ cup thinly sliced green or black olives

- 4 Tbsp. 2% reduced-fat plain Greek yogurt

- Juice of 1 lemon

- 2 tsp fresh chopped dill

- 1 Tbsp. fresh chopped oregano

- ½ tsp smoked paprika

- ½ tsp sea salt

- ¼ tsp black pepper

- 1 cup dry farro

Directions:

1. In a bowl, add the olive oil, garlic, lemon, dill, oregano, paprika, salt, and pepper, whisk to combine

2. Pour 3/4 the amount of marinade over shrimp, toss to coat and all to stand 10 minutes

3. Reserve the rest of the marinade for later

4. Cook the farro according to package instructions in water or chicken stock

5. In a grill pan or nonstick skillet over medium heat, add the olive

6. Once heated, add shrimp, cook for 2-3 minutes per side, until no longer pink, then transfer to a plate

7. Working in batches, cook bell pepper, zucchinis, and cherry tomatoes to the grill pan or skillet, cook for 5-6 minutes, until softened

8. allow the dish to cool completely

9. Distribute the farro among the containers, evenly add the shrimp, grilled vegetables, olives, and tomatoes, store for 2 days

10. To Serve: Reheat in the microwave for 1-2 minutes or until heated through. Drizzle the reserved marinade over top. Top each bowl with 1 tbsp Greek yogurt and extra lemon juice, if desired

Nutrition Info:Per Serving: Calories:428;Carbs: 45g;Total Fat: 13g;Protein: 34g

Asparagus Salmon Fillets

Servings: 2

Cooking Time: 30 Minutes

Ingredients:

- 1 teaspoon olive oil

- 4 asparagus stalks

- 2 salmon fillets

- ¼ cup butter

- ¼ cup champagne

- Salt and freshly ground black pepper, to taste

Directions:

1. Preheat the oven to 355 degrees F and grease a baking dish.

2. Put all the ingredients in a bowl and mix well.

101

3. Put this mixture in the baking dish and transfer it in the oven.

4. Bake for about 20 minutes and dish out.

5. Place the salmon fillets in a dish and keep aside to cool for meal prepping. Divide it into 2 containers and close the lid. Refrigerate for 1 day and reheat in microwave before serving.

Nutrition Info: Calories: 475 ;Carbohydrates: 1.1g;Protein: 35.2g;Fat: 38g;Sugar: 0.5g;Sodium: 242mg

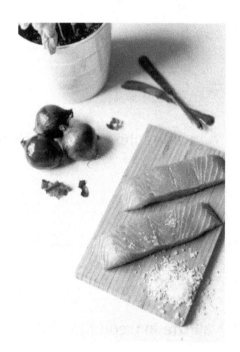

Grilled Calamari With Berries

Servings: 4

Cooking Time: 5 Minutes

Ingredients:

- ¼ cup olive oil

- ¼ cup extra virgin olive oil

- 1 thinly sliced apple

- ¾ cup blueberries

- ¼ cup sliced almonds

- 1 ½ pounds calamari tube

- ¼ cup dried cranberries

- 6 cups spinach

- 2 tablespoons apple cider vinegar

- 1 tablespoon lemon juice

- Sea salt and pepper to your liking

Directions:

1. Start by making the vinaigrette. Combine apple cider vinegar, lemon juice, extra virgin olive oil, sea salt, and pepper. Whisk well and set aside.

2. Set your grill to medium heat.

3. In a separate bowl, add the calamari tube and mix with salt, pepper, and olive oil.

4. Set the calamari on the grill and cook both sides for 2 to 3 minutes.

5. In another bowl, mix the salad by adding the spinach, cranberries, almonds, blueberries, and apples. Toss to mix.

6. Set the cooked calamari onto a cutting board and let it cool for a few minutes. Cut them into

¼-inch thick rings and then toss them into the salad bowl.

7. Sprinkle the vinaigrette sauce onto the salad. Toss to mix the ingredients and enjoy!

Nutrition Info: calories: 567, fats: 24.4 grams, carbohydrates: 30 grams, protein: 55 grams.

Italian Sausage And Veggie Pizza Pasta

Servings: 8

Cooking Time: 30 Minutes

Ingredients:

- 1 tsp olive oil

- 1 (2.25 oz) can of sliced black olives

- 1 (28 oz) can of tomato sauce

- 1 (16 oz) box penne pasta

- 3 cups water

- 3 sweet Italian sausage links, casings removed, around 1 lb of sausage

- 1 cup sliced onions

- 1 cup sliced green bell pepper

- 2-3 garlic cloves, minced or pressed

- 8 oz. sliced mushrooms

- 1/2 cup Pepperoni, cut in half and then each half cut into thirds + a few extra whole pieces for topping

- 1/2 tsp Italian seasoning

- 1/2 tsp salt

- Salt, to taste

- Pepper to taste

- 2 cups shredded mozzarella cheese, divided

- Garnish:

- Chopped fresh parsley and Romano cheese

Directions:

1. In a deep heavy-bottom, oven-safe pot over medium heat, add the oil

2. Once heated, add in the sausage and break it up with a wooden spoon

3. Then add in the onions, peppers, garlic and mushrooms, stir to combine, season with salt and pepper to taste. Sauté until the sausage crumbles have browned, stirring frequently for around 10 minutes

4. Add in the pepperoni and olives to the pan, sauté for 1-2 minutes.

5. Then add in the sauce, water, Italian seasoning, salt and pasta to the pan, stir to combine

6. Bring the pot to a boil

7. Once boiling, reduce the heat to medium low, cover and allow to simmer for 10 minutes, stirring occasionally

8. Remove the cover and continue to simmer for 3-5 minutes, stirring occasionally

9. Stir in 1/2 cup of shredded Mozzarella cheese, sprinkle the remaining cheese on top

10. Arrange a few more whole pepperonis on top of the cheese, broil for a few minutes until the cheese is bubbling and melted

11. Top with the parsley and Romano cheese

12. Allow to cool and distribute the pasta evenly among the containers. Store in the fridge for 3-4 days or in the freezer for 2 weeks.

13. To Serve: Reheat in the oven at 375 degrees for 1-2 minutes or until heated through.

14. Recipe Note: If you would like it to be spicy, you can also use hot Italian sausage.

Nutrition Info:Per Serving: Calories:450;Total Fat: 21.9g;Total Carbs: 22g;Fiber: 5g;Protein: 43g

Baked Chicken Thighs With Lemon, Olives, And Brussels Sprouts

Servings: 4

Cooking Time: 40 Minutes

Ingredients:

- 2 tablespoons olive oil, divided

- 1 pound Brussels sprouts, stemmed and halved (quartered if the sprouts are extra large)

- 1 pound boneless, skinless chicken thighs

- 2 teaspoons chopped garlic

- 1 teaspoon dried oregano

- ½ teaspoon kosher salt

- 3 tablespoons freshly squeezed lemon juice

- ½ cup pitted kalamata olives

Directions:

1. Preheat the oven to 350°F.

2. Spread 1 tablespoon of oil over the bottom of a 13-by-9-inch glass or ceramic baking dish. Add the Brussels sprouts to the pan and spread out evenly. Place the chicken on top of the sprouts and rub the garlic and oregano into the top of the chicken.

3. Sprinkle the salt, the remaining 1 tablespoon of oil, the lemon juice, and the olives over the contents of the pan.

4. Cover the pan with aluminum foil and bake for 20 minutes. Remove the foil and bake uncovered for 20 more minutes. Cool.

5. Place one quarter of the chicken and ¾ cup of Brussels sprouts in each of 4 containers. Drizzle any remaining juices from the pan over the chicken.

6. STORAGE: Store covered containers in the refrigerator for 5 days.

Nutrition Info:Per Serving: Total calories: 28 Total fat: 18g; Saturated fat: 3g; Sodium: 737mg; Carbohydrates: 14g; Fiber: 5g; Protein: 20g

Slow Cooker Lamb, Herb, And Bean Stew

Servings: 4

Cooking Time: 15 Minutes

Ingredients:

- 3 bunches of parsley (about 6 packed cups of leaves)

- 1 large bunch cilantro (about 1½ packed cups of leaves)

- 1 bunch scallions, sliced (both white and green parts, about 1¼ cups)

- 1 pound leg of lamb, fat trimmed, cut into 1-inch pieces

- 2 tablespoons olive oil, divided

- 1 medium onion, chopped

- 2 teaspoons chopped garlic

- 2 teaspoons turmeric

- ¾ teaspoon kosher salt

- 2 tablespoons tomato paste

- 2½ cups low-sodium chicken broth

- 2 (15.5-ounce) cans low-sodium kidney beans, drained and rinsed

- 2 tablespoons freshly squeezed lemon juice

Directions:

1. Finely chop the parsley leaves, cilantro leaves, and scallions with a knife, or pulse in the food processor until finely chopped but not puréed. With this amount of herbs, you'll need to pulse in two batches.

2. Pat the lamb cubes with a paper towel. Heat a 1inch skillet over medium-high heat and add 1 tablespoon of oil. Once the oil is shimmering,

add the lamb and brown for 5 minutes, flipping after 3 minutes. Place the lamb in the slow cooker.

3. Turn the heat down to medium and add the remaining 1 tablespoon of oil to the skillet. Once the oil is hot, add the onions and garlic and sauté for minutes. Add the turmeric, salt, and tomato paste and continue to cook for 2 more minutes, stirring frequently.

4. Add the chopped parsley, cilantro, and scallions. Sauté for 5 minutes, stirring occasionally.

5. While the herbs are cooking, add the broth, beans, and lemon juice to the slow cooker. Add the herb mixture when it's done cooking on the stove. Turn the slow cooker to the low setting and cook for 8 hours.

6. Taste and add more salt and/or lemon juice if needed. Cool.

7. Scoop 2 cups of stew into each of 4 containers.

8. STORAGE: Store covered containers in the refrigerator for up to 5 days. Stew can be frozen for up to 4 months.

Nutrition Info:Per Serving: Total calories: 486; Total fat: 15g; Saturated fat: 5g; Sodium: 6mg; Carbohydrates: 51g; Fiber: 15g; Protein: 41g

Holiday Chicken Salad

Servings: 2

Cooking Time: 25 Minutes

Ingredients:

- 1 celery stalk, chopped

- 1½ cups cooked grass-fed chicken, chopped

- ¼ cup fresh cranberries

- ¼ cup sour cream

- ½ apple, chopped

- ¼ yellow onion, chopped

- 1/8 cup almonds, toasted and chopped

- 2-ounce feta cheese, crumbled

- ¼ cup avocado mayonnaise

- Salt and black pepper, to taste

Directions:

1. Stir together all the ingredients in a bowl except almonds and cheese.

2. Top with almonds and cheese to serve.

3. Meal Prep Tip: Don't add almonds and cheese in the salad if you want to store the salad. Cover with a plastic wrap and refrigerate to serve.

Nutrition Info: Calories: 336 ;Carbohydrates: 8.8g;Protein: 25g;Fat: 23.2g ;Sugar: 5.4g;Sodium: 383mg

Costa Brava Chicken

Servings: 4

Cooking Time: 35 Minutes

Ingredients:

- 1 20-ounce can pineapple chunks

- 10 skinless and boneless chicken breast halves

- 1 tablespoon vegetable oil

- 1 teaspoon ground cumin

- 1 teaspoon ground cinnamon

- 2garlic cloves, minced

- 1 onion, quartered

- 1 14-ounce can stewed tomatoes

- 2 cups black olives

- ½ cup salsa

- 2 tablespoons water

- 1 red bell pepper, thinly sliced

- salt

Directions:

1. Drain the pineapple chunks, but be sure to reserve the juice.

2. Sprinkle pineapples with salt.

3. Heat oil in a large frying pan over medium heat.

4. Add the chicken and cook until brown.

5. Combine the cinnamon and cumin and sprinkle over the chicken.

6. Add garlic and onion and cook until the onions are tender.

7. Add reserved pineapple juices, olives, tomatoes, and salsa.

8. Reduce heat, cover, and allow to simmer for 25 minutes.

9. Combine the cornstarch and water in a bowl.

10. Add the cornstarch mixture to the pan and stir.

11. Add the bell pepper and simmer for a little longer until the sauce bubbles and thickens.

12. Stir in pineapple chunks until thoroughly heated.

13. Enjoy!

Nutrition Info:Per Serving: Calories: 651, Total Fat: 16.5 g, Saturated Fat: 1.7 g, Cholesterol: 228 mg, Sodium: 1053 mg, Total Carbohydrate: 34.7 g, Dietary Fiber: 7.2 g, Total Sugars: 20.3 g, Protein: 94.5 g, Vitamin D: 0 mcg, Calcium: 118 mg, Iron: 6 mg, Potassium: 606 mg

One Skillet Greek Lemon Chicken And Rice

Servings: 5

Cooking Time: 45 Minutes

Ingredients:

- Marinade:

- 2 tsp dried oregano

- 1 tsp dried minced onion

- 4-5 cloves garlic, minced

- Zest of 1 lemon

- 1/2 tsp kosher salt

- 1/2 tsp black pepper

- 1-2 Tbsp olive oil to make a loose paste

- 5 bone-in, skin on chicken thighs

- Rice:

- 1 1/2 Tbsp olive oil

- 1 large yellow onion, peeled and diced

- 1 cup dry long-grain white rice (NOT minute or quick cooking varieties)

- 2 cups chicken stock

- 1 1/4 tsp dried oregano

- 5 cloves garlic, minced

- 3/4 tsp kosher salt

- 1/2 tsp black pepper

- Lemon slices, optional

- Fresh minced parsley, for garnish

- Extra lemon zest, for garnish

Directions:

1. In a large resealable plastic bag, add the oregano, dried minced onion, garlic, lemon zest, salt, black pepper, and olive oil, massage to combine

2. Add chicken thighs, and then turn/massage to coat, refrigerate 15 minutes or overnight

3. Preheat oven to 0 F degrees

4. In a large cast iron or heavy oven safe skillet over medium-high heat, add 1 1/2 Tbsp olive oil to

5. Remove the chicken thighs from the refrigerator, shake off the excess marinade and add chicken thighs, skin side down, to pan, cook 4-minutes per side

6. Transfer to a plate and wipe the skillet lightly with a paper towel to remove any burnt bits, reserving chicken grease in pan.

7. Lower the heat to medium and add onion to pan, cook 3-4 minutes, until softened and slightly charred. Add in garlic and cook 1 minute

8. Then add in the rice, oregano, salt and pepper, stir together and cook for 1 minute

9. Pour in chicken stock, turn the temperature up to medium-high, bring to a simmer

10. Once simmering, place the chicken thighs on top of the rice mixture, push down gently

11. Cover with lid or foil, and bake 35 minutes

12. Uncover, return to oven and bake an additional 10-15 minutes, until liquid is removed, the rice is tender, and chicken is cooked through

13. Allow the rice and chicken to cool

14. Distribute among the containers, store in fridge for 2-3 days

15. To serve: Reheat in the microwave for 1 minute to 2 minutes or cooked through. Garnish with lemon zest and parsley, and serve!

Nutrition Info:Per Serving: Calories:325;Carbs: 35g;Total Fat: 11g;Protein: 21g

Trout With Wilted Greens

Servings: 4

Cooking Time: 15 Minutes

Ingredients:

- 2 teaspoons extra virgin olive oil

- 2 cups kale, chopped

- 2 cups Swiss chard, chopped

- ½ sweet onion, thinly sliced

- 4 (5 ounce boneless skin-on trout fillets)

- Juice of 1 lemon

- Sea salt

- Freshly ground pepper

- Zest of 1 lemon

Directions:

1. Pre-heat your oven to 375-degree Fahrenheit

2. Lightly grease a 9 by 13-inch baking dish with olive oil

3. Arrange the kale, Swiss chard, onion in a dish

4. Top greens with fish, skin side up and drizzle with olive oil and lemon juice

5. Season fish with salt and pepper

6. Bake for 15 minutes until fish flakes

7. Sprinkle zest

8. Serve and enjoy!

9. Meal Prep/Storage Options: Store in airtight containers in your fridge for 1-3 days.

Nutrition Info: Calories: 315;Fat: 14g;Carbohydrates: 6g;Protein: 39g

One Skillet Chicken In Roasted Red Pepper Sauce

Servings: 4

Cooking Time: 20 Minutes

Ingredients:

- 4-6 boneless skinless chicken thighs or breasts

- 2/3 cup chopped roasted red peppers (see note)

- 2 tsp Italian seasoning, divided

- 4 tbsp oil

- 1 tbsp minced garlic

- 1/2 tsp salt

- 1/4 tsp black pepper

- 1 cup heavy cream

- 2 tbsp crumbled feta cheese, optional

- Thinly sliced fresh basil, optional

Directions:

1. In a blender or food processer, combine the roasted red peppers, tsp Italian seasoning, oil, garlic, salt, and pepper, pulse until smooth.

2. In a large skillet over medium heat, add the olive oil and season chicken with remaining 1 tsp Italian seasoning. Cook chicken for 6-8 minutes on each side, or until cooked through and lightly browned on the outside. Then transfer to a plate and cover

3. Add the red pepper mixture to the pan, stir over medium heat 2-minutes, or until heated throughout. Add the heavy cream, stir until mixture is thick and creamy

4. Add chicken, toss in the sauce to coat

5. allow the dish to cool completely

6. Distribute among the containers, store for 2-3 days

7. To Serve: Reheat in the microwave for 1-2 minutes or until heated through. Garnish with crumbled feta cheese and fresh basil. Serve with your favorite grain.

8. Recipe Notes: You can purchase jarred roasted red peppers at most grocery stores around the olives.

Nutrition Info:Per Serving: Calories:655;Carbs: 12g;Total Fat: 25g;Protein: 8

Mediterranean Minestrone Soup

Servings: 4

Cooking Time: 40 Minutes

Ingredients:

- 1 large onion, finely chopped

- 4 cups vegetable stock

- 4 cloves crushed garlic

- 1 ounce chopped carrots

- 4 ounces chopped red bell pepper

- 4 ounces chopped celery (keep leaves)

- 1 16-ounce can diced tomatoes

- 1 16-ounce can white beans

- 4 ounces fresh spinach, chopped

- 4 ounces multi-colored pasta

- 2 ounces grated parmesan

- 2 tablespoons olive oil

- bunch of chopped parsley

- 1 teaspoon dried oregano

- salt

- pepper

- 4 ounces salami, finely sliced (if desired)

Directions:

1. Heat oil in a pan over medium heat.

2. Add chopped onions, red pepper, carrots, and celery.

3. Saute for about 10 minutes until tender.

4. Add garlic and cook on low heat for 2 minutes more.

5. Add your stock and tomatoes and cook for an additional 10 minutes.

6. Add pasta and cook for 15 minutes more until al dente.

7. Taste / check your seasoning; add salt and pepper as needed.

8. Add parsley, beans, celery leaves, spinach, and salami (if using), and stir.

9. Pour the whole mixture to a boil and stir for about 2 minutes.

10. Enjoy the soup hot!

Nutrition Info:Per Serving: Calories: 888, Total Fat: 19.9 g, Saturated Fat: 6.3 g, Cholesterol: 30 mg, Sodium: 1200 mg, Total Carbohydrate: 139.5 g, Dietary Fiber: 31.8 g, Total Sugars: 14.3 g, Protein:

49.4 g, Vitamin D: 14 mcg, Calcium: 64.3 mg, Iron: 22 mg, Potassium: 3951 mg

Baked Shrimp Stew

Servings: 4-6

Cooking Time: 25 Minutes

Ingredients:

- Greek extra virgin olive oil

- 2 1/2 lb prawns, peeled, deveined, rinsed well and dried

- 1 large red onion, chopped (about two cups)

- 5 garlic cloves, roughly chopped

- 1 red bell pepper, seeded, chopped

- 2 15-oz cans diced tomatoes

- 1/2 cup water

- 1 1/2 tsp ground coriander

- 1 tsp sumac

- 1 tsp cumin

- 1 tsp red pepper flakes, more to taste

- 1/2 tsp ground green cardamom

- Salt and pepper, to taste

- 1 cup parsley leaves, stems removed

- 1/3 cup toasted pine nuts

- 1/4 cup toasted sesame seeds

- Lemon or lime wedges to serve

Directions:

1. Preheat the oven to 375 degrees F

2. In a large frying pan, add 1 tbsp olive oil

3. Sauté the prawns for 2 minutes, until they are barely pink, then remove and set aside

4. In the same pan over medium-high heat, drizzle a little more olive oil and sauté the chopped onions, garlic and red bell peppers for 5 minutes, stirring regularly

5. Add in the canned diced tomatoes and water, allow to simmer for 10 minutes, until the liquid reduces, stir occasionally

6. Reduce the heat to medium, add the shrimp back to the pan, stir in the spices the ground coriander, sumac, cumin, red pepper flakes, green cardamom, salt and pepper, then the toasted pine nuts, sesame seeds and parsley leaves, stir to combined

7. Transfer the shrimp and sauce to an oven-safe earthenware or stoneware dish, cover tightly with foil Place in the oven to bake for minutes, uncover and broil briefly.

8. allow the dish to cool completely

9. Distribute among the containers, store for 2-3 days

10. To Serve: Reheat on the stove for 1-2 minutes or until heated through. Serve with your favorite bread or whole grain. Garnish with a side of lime or lemon wedges.

Nutrition Info:Per Serving: Calories:377;Carbs: ;Total Fat: 20g;Protein: 41g

Rainbow Salad With Roasted Chickpeas

Servings: 2-3

Cooking Time: 40 Minutes

Ingredients:

- Creamy avocado dressing, store bought or homemade

- 3 large tri-color carrots - one orange, one red, and one yellow

- 1 medium zucchini

- 1/4 cup fresh basil, cut into ribbons

- 1 can chickpeas, rinsed and drained

- 1 tbsp olive oil

- 1 tsp chili powder

- 1/2 tsp cumin

- Salt, to taste

- Pepper, to taste

Directions:

1. Preheat the oven to 400 degrees F

2. Pat the chickpeas dry with paper towels

3. Add them to a bowl and toss with the olive oil, chili powder, cumin, and salt and pepper

4. Arrange the chickpeas on a baking sheet in a single layer

5. Bake for 30-40 minutes - making sure to shaking the pan once in a while to prevent over browning. The chickpeas will be done when they're crispy and golden brown, allow to cool

6. With a grater, peeler, mandolin or spiralizer, shred the carrots and zucchini into very thin ribbons

7. Once the zucchini is shredded, lightly press it with paper towels to remove excess moisture

8. Add the shredded zucchini and carrots to a bowl, toss with the basil

9. Add in the roasted chickpeas, too gently to combine

10. Distribute among the containers, store for 2 days

11. To Serve: Top with the avocado dressing and enjoy

Nutrition Info:Per Serving: (without dressing): Calories:640;Total Fat: 51g;Total Carbs: 9.8g;Protein: 38.8g

Sour And Sweet Fish

Servings: 2

Cooking Time: 25 Minutes

Ingredients:

- 1 tablespoon vinegar

- 2 drops stevia

- 1 pound fish chunks

- ¼ cup butter, melted

- Salt and black pepper, to taste

Directions:

1. Put butter and fish chunks in a skillet and cook for about 3 minutes.

2. Add stevia, salt and black pepper and cook for about 10 minutes, stirring continuously.

3. Dish out in a bowl and serve immediately.

4. Place fish in a dish and set aside to cool for meal prepping. Divide it in 2 containers and refrigerate for up to 2 days. Reheat in microwave before serving.

Nutrition Info: Calories: 2 ;Carbohydrates: 2.8g;Protein: 24.5g;Fat: 16.7g;Sugar: 2.7g;Sodium: 649mg

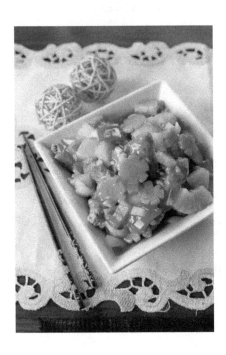

Papaya Mangetout Stew

Servings: 2

Cooking Time: 5 Minutes

Ingredients:

- 2 cups Mangetout

- 2 cups bean sprouts

- 1 tablespoon water

- 1 papaya, peeled, deseeded, and cubed

- 1 lime, juiced

- 2 tablespoon unsalted peanuts

- small handful basil leaves, torn

- small handful mint leaves, chopped

Directions:

1. Take a large frying pan and place it over high heat.

2. Add Mangetout, 1 tablespoon of water, and bean sprouts.

3. Cook for about 2-minutes.

4. Remove from heat, add papaya, and lime juice.

5. Toss everything well.

6. Spread over containers.

7. Before eating, garnish with herbs and peanuts.

8. Enjoy!

Nutrition Info:Per Serving: Calories: 283, Total Fat: 6.4 g, Saturated Fat: 0.g, Cholesterol: 0 mg, Sodium: 148 mg, Total Carbohydrate: 42.8 g, Dietary Fiber: 4.9 g, Total Sugars: 21.5 g, Protein: 20.1 g, Vitamin D: 0 mcg, Calcium: 205 mg, Iron: 3 mg, Potassium: 743 mg

Mediterranean Pork Pita Sandwich

Servings: 6

Cooking Time: 10 Minutes

Ingredients:

- 2 teaspoons olive oil, plus 1 tablespoon

- 2 cups packed baby spinach leaves, finely chopped

- 4 ounces mushrooms, finely chopped

- 1 teaspoon chopped garlic

- 1 pound extra-lean ground pork

- 1 large egg

- ½ cup panko bread crumbs

- ⅓ cup chopped fresh dill

- ¼ teaspoon kosher salt

- 6 large romaine lettuce leaves, ripped into pieces to fit pita

- 2 tomatoes, sliced

- 3 whole-wheat pitas, cut in half

- ¾ cup Garlic Yogurt Sauce

Directions:

1. Heat 2 teaspoons of oil in a -inch skillet over medium heat. Once the oil is shimmering, add the spinach, mushrooms, and garlic and sauté for 3 minutes. Cool for 5 minutes.

2. Place the mushroom mixture in a large mixing bowl and add the pork, egg, bread crumbs, dill, and salt. Mix with your hands until everything is well combined. Make 6 patties, about ½-inch thick and 3 inches in diameter.

3. Heat the remaining 1 tablespoon of oil in the same 12-inch skillet over medium-high heat. When the oil is hot, add the patties. They

should all be able to fit in the pan. If not, cook in 2 batches. Cook for 5 minutes on the first side and 4 minutes on the second side. The outside should be golden brown, and the inside should no longer be pink.

4. Place 1 patty in each of 6 containers. In each of 6 separate containers that will not be reheated, place 1 torn lettuce leaf and 2 tomato slices. Wrap the pita halves in plastic wrap and place one in each veggie container. Spoon 2 tablespoons of yogurt sauce into each of 6 sauce containers.

5. STORAGE: Store covered containers in the refrigerator for up to days. Uncooked patties can be frozen for up to 4 months, while cooked patties can be frozen for up to 3 months.

Nutrition Info:Per Serving: Total calories: 309; Total fat: 11g; Saturated fat: 3g; Sodium: 343mg; Carbohydrates: 22g; Fiber: 3g; Protein: 32g

Salmon With Warm Tomato-olive Salad

Servings: 4

Cooking Time: 25 Minutes

Ingredients:

- Salmon fillets (4/approx. 4 oz./1.25-inches thick)

- Celery (1 cup)

- Medium tomatoes (2)

- Fresh mint (.25 cup)

- Kalamata olives (.5 cup)

- Garlic (.5 tsp.)

- Salt (1 tsp. + more to taste)

- Honey (1 tbsp.)

- Red pepper flakes (.25 tsp.)

- Olive oil (2 tbsp. + more for the pan)

- Vinegar (1 tsp.)

Directions:

1. Slice the tomatoes and celery into inch pieces and mince the garlic. Chop the mint and the olives.

2. Heat the oven using the broiler setting.

3. Whisk the oil, vinegar, honey, red pepper flakes, and salt (1 tsp.. Brush the mixture onto the salmon.

4. Line the broiler pan with a sheet of foil. Spritz the pan lightly with olive oil, and add the fillets (skin side downward.

5. Broil them for four to six minutes until well done.

6. Meanwhile, make the tomato salad. Mix ½ teaspoon of the salt with the garlic.

7. Prepare a small saucepan on the stovetop using the med-high temperature setting. Pour in the rest of the oil and add the garlic mixture with the olives and one tablespoon of vinegar. Simmer for about three minutes.

8. Prepare the serving dishes. Pour the bubbly mixture into the bowl and add the mint, tomato, and celery. Dust it with the salt as desired and toss.

9. When the salmon is done, serve with a tomato salad.

Nutrition Info: Calories: 433;Protein: 38 grams;Fat: 26 grams

Conclusion

We've reached the end of this book, and after delighting in wonderful candlelight dinners, we can now see how much we enjoyed these delicious dishes.

Did your family enjoy them?

Did you win over the woman or man in your life?

Keep practicing with these delicious dishes and you'll be great!

Hugs to you and thank you.